INDIAN COOKBOOK 2021

EASY TO MAKE RECIPES FROM THE INDIAN TRADITION

SECOND EDITION

NATHALIE BROWN

Table of Contents

Zunka

(Spicy Gram Flour Curry)

Serves 4

Ingredients

750g/1lb 10oz besan*, dry roasted

400ml/14fl oz water

4 tbsp refined vegetable oil

½ tsp mustard seeds

½ tsp cumin seeds

½ tsp turmeric

3-4 green chillies, slit lengthways

10 garlic cloves, crushed

3 small onions, finely chopped

1 tsp tamarind paste

Salt to taste

Method

- Mix the besan with enough water to form a thick paste. Set aside.

- Heat the oil in a saucepan. Add the mustard and cumin seeds. Let them splutter for 15 seconds. Add the remaining ingredients. Fry for a minute. Add the besan paste and stir continuously on a low heat till thick. Serve hot.

Turnip Curry

Serves 4

Ingredients

3 tsp poppy seeds

3 tsp sesame seeds

3 tsp coriander seeds

3 tsp fresh coconut, grated

125g/4½oz yoghurt

120ml/4fl oz refined vegetable oil

2 large onions, finely chopped

1½ tsp chilli powder

1 tsp ginger paste

1 tsp garlic paste

400g/14oz turnips, chopped

Salt to taste

Method

- Dry roast the poppy, sesame and coriander seeds and the coconut for 1-2 minutes. Grind to a paste.

- Whisk this paste with the yoghurt. Set aside.

- Heat the oil in a saucepan. Add the remaining ingredients. Fry them on a medium heat for 5 minutes. Add the yoghurt mixture. Simmer for 7-8 minutes. Serve hot.

Chhaner Dhalna

(Bengali Style Paneer)

Serves 4

Ingredients

2 tbsp mustard oil plus extra for deep frying

225g/8oz paneer*, diced

2.5cm/1in cinnamon

3 green cardamom pods

4 cloves

½ tsp cumin seeds

1 tsp turmeric

2 large potatoes, diced and fried

½ tsp chilli powder

2 tsp sugar

Salt to taste

250ml/8fl oz water

2 tbsp coriander leaves, chopped

Method

- Heat the oil for deep frying in a frying pan. Add the paneer and fry on a medium heat till golden brown. Drain and set aside.

- Heat the remaining oil in a saucepan. Add the remaining ingredients, except the water and coriander leaves. Fry for 2-3 minutes.

- Add the water. Simmer for 7-8 minutes. Add the paneer. Simmer for 5 more minutes. Garnish with the coriander leaves. Serve hot.

Corn with Coconut

Serves 4

Ingredients

2 tbsp ghee

600g/1lb 5oz corn kernels, cooked

1 tsp sugar

1 tsp salt

10g/¼oz coriander leaves, finely chopped

For the coconut paste:

50g/1¾oz fresh coconut, grated

3 tbsp poppy seeds

1 tsp coriander seeds

2.5cm/1in root ginger, julienned

3 green chillies

125g/4½oz peanuts

Method

- Coarsely grind all the ingredients for the coconut paste. Heat the ghee in a frying pan. Add the paste and fry for 4-5 minutes, stirring continuously.

- Add the corn, sugar and salt. Cook on a low heat for 4-5 minutes.

- Garnish with the coriander leaves. Serve hot.

Green Pepper with Potato

Serves 4

Ingredients

2 tbsp refined vegetable oil

1 tsp cumin seeds

10 garlic cloves, finely chopped

3 large potatoes, diced

2 tsp ground coriander

1 tsp ground cumin

½ tsp turmeric

½ tsp amchoor*

½ tsp garam masala

Salt to taste

3 large green peppers, julienned

3 tbsp coriander leaves, chopped

Method

- Heat the oil in a saucepan. Add the cumin seeds and garlic. Fry for 30 seconds.

- Add the remaining ingredients, except the peppers and coriander leaves. Stir-fry on a medium heat for 5-6 minutes.

- Add the peppers. Stir-fry on a low heat for 5 more minutes. Garnish with the coriander leaves. Serve hot.

Spicy Peas with Potatoes

Serves 4

Ingredients

2 tbsp refined vegetable oil

1 tsp ginger paste

1 large onion, finely chopped

2 large potatoes, diced

500g/1lb 2oz canned peas

½ tsp turmeric

Salt to taste

½ tsp garam masala

2 large tomatoes, diced

½ tsp chilli powder

1 tsp sugar

1 tbsp coriander leaves, chopped

Method

- Heat the oil in a saucepan. Add the ginger paste and onion. Fry them till the onion is translucent.

- Add the remaining ingredients, except the coriander leaves. Mix well. Cover with a lid and cook on a low heat for 10 minutes.

- Garnish with the coriander leaves. Serve hot.

Sautéed Mushrooms

Ingredients

2 tbsp refined vegetable oil

4 green chillies, slit lengthways

8 garlic cloves, crushed

100g/3½oz green peppers, sliced

400g/14oz mushrooms, sliced

Salt to taste

½ tsp coarsely ground black pepper

25g/scant 1oz coriander leaves, chopped

Method

- Heat the oil in a frying pan. Add the green chillies, garlic and green peppers. Fry them on a medium heat for 1-2 minutes.

- Add the mushrooms, salt and pepper. Mix well. Sauté on a medium heat till tender. Garnish with the coriander leaves. Serve hot.

Spicy Mushroom with Baby Corn

Serves 4

Ingredients

2 tbsp refined vegetable oil

1 tsp cumin seeds

2 bay leaves

1 tsp ginger paste

2 green chillies, finely chopped

1 large onion, finely chopped

200g/7oz mushrooms, halved

8-10 baby corns, chopped

125g/4½oz tomato purée

½ tsp turmeric

Salt to taste

½ tsp garam masala

½ tsp sugar

10g/¼oz coriander leaves, chopped

Method

- Heat the oil in a saucepan. Add the cumin seeds and bay leaves. Let them splutter for 15 seconds.

- Add the ginger paste, green chillies and onion. Sauté for 1-2 minutes.

- Add the remaining ingredients, except the coriander leaves. Mix well. Cover with a lid and cook on a low heat for 10 minutes.

- Garnish with the coriander leaves. Serve hot.

Dry Spicy Cauliflower

Serves 4

Ingredients

750g/1lb 10oz cauliflower florets

Salt to taste

Pinch of turmeric

4 bay leaves

750ml/1¼ pints water

2 tbsp refined vegetable oil

4 cloves

4 green cardamom pods

1 large onion, sliced

1 tsp ginger paste

1 tsp garlic paste

1 tsp garam masala

½ tsp chilli powder

¼ tsp ground black pepper

10 cashew nuts, ground

2 tbsp yoghurt

3 tbsp tomato purée

3 tbsp butter

60ml/2fl oz single cream

Method

- Cook the cauliflower with the salt, turmeric, bay leaves and water in a saucepan on a medium heat for 10 minutes. Drain and arrange the florets in an ovenproof dish. Set aside.

- Heat the oil in a saucepan. Add the cloves and cardamom. Let them splutter for 15 seconds.

- Add the onion, ginger paste and garlic paste. Fry for a minute.

- Add the garam masala, chilli powder, pepper and cashew nuts. Fry for 1-2 minutes.

- Add the yoghurt and tomato purée. Mix thoroughly. Add the butter and cream. Stir for a minute. Remove from the heat.

- Pour this over the cauliflower florets. Bake at 150°C (300°F, Gas Mark 2) in a pre-heated oven for 8-10 minutes. Serve hot.

Mushroom Curry

Serves 4

Ingredients

3 tbsp refined vegetable oil

2 large onions, grated

1 tsp ginger paste

1 tsp garlic paste

½ tsp turmeric

1 tsp chilli powder

1 tsp ground coriander

400g/14oz mushrooms, quartered

200g/7oz peas

2 tomatoes, finely chopped

½ tsp garam masala

Salt to taste

20 cashew nuts, ground

240ml/6fl oz water

Method

- Heat the oil in a saucepan. Add the onions. Fry them till they are brown.

- Add the ginger paste, garlic paste, turmeric, chilli powder and ground coriander. Sauté on a medium heat for a minute.

- Add the remaining ingredients. Mix well. Cover with a lid and simmer for 8-10 minutes. Serve hot.

Baingan Bharta

(Roasted Aubergine)

Serves 4

Ingredients

1 large aubergine

3 tbsp refined vegetable oil

1 large onion, finely chopped

3 green chillies, slit lengthways

¼ tsp turmeric

Salt to taste

½ tsp garam masala

1 tomato, finely chopped

Method

- Pierce the aubergine all over with a fork and grill it for 25 minutes. Once it has cooled, discard the roasted skin and mash the flesh. Set aside.

- Heat the oil in a saucepan. Add the onion and green chillies. Fry on a medium heat for 2 minutes.

- Add the turmeric, salt, garam masala and tomato. Mix well. Fry for 5 minutes. Add the mashed aubergine. Mix well.

- Cook on a low heat for 8 minutes, stirring occasionally. Serve hot.

Vegetable Hyderabadi

Serves 4

Ingredients

2 tbsp refined vegetable oil

½ tsp mustard seeds

1 large onion, finely chopped

400g/14oz frozen, mixed vegetables

½ tsp turmeric

Salt to taste

For the spice mixture:

2.5cm/1in root ginger

8 garlic cloves

2 cloves

2.5cm/1in cinnamon

1 tsp fenugreek seeds

3 green chillies

4 tbsp fresh coconut, grated

10 cashew nuts

Method

- Grind all the ingredients of the spice mixture together. Set aside.

- Heat the oil in a saucepan. Add the mustard seeds. Let them splutter for 15 seconds. Add the onion and fry till brown.

- Add the remaining ingredients and the ground spice mixture. Mix well. Cook on a low heat for 8-10 minutes. Serve hot.

Kaddu Bhaji*

(Dry Red Pumpkin)

Serves 4

Ingredients

3 tbsp refined vegetable oil

½ tsp cumin seeds

¼ tsp fenugreek seeds

600g/1lb 5oz pumpkin, thinly sliced

Salt to taste

½ tsp roasted ground cumin

½ tsp chilli powder

¼ tsp turmeric

1 tsp amchoor*

1 tsp sugar

Method

- Heat the oil in a saucepan. Add the cumin and fenugreek seeds. Let them splutter for 15 seconds. Add the pumpkin and salt. Mix well. Cover with a lid and cook on a medium heat for 8 minutes.

- Uncover and lightly crush with the back of a spoon. Add the remaining ingredients. Mix well. Cook for 5 minutes. Serve hot.

Muthia nu Shak

(Fenugreek Dumplings in Sauce)

Serves 4

Ingredients

200g/7oz fresh fenugreek leaves, finely chopped

Salt to taste

125g/4½oz wholemeal flour

125g/4½oz besan*

2 green chillies, finely chopped

1 tsp ginger paste

3 tsp sugar

Juice of 1 lemon

½ tsp garam masala

½ tsp turmeric

Pinch of bicarbonate of soda

3 tbsp refined vegetable oil

½ tsp ajowan seeds

½ tsp mustard seeds

Pinch of asafoetida

250ml/8fl oz water

Method

- Mix the fenugreek leaves with the salt. Set aside for 10 minutes. Squeeze out the moisture.

- Mix the fenugreek leaves with the flour, besan, green chillies, ginger paste, sugar, lemon juice, garam masala, turmeric and bicarbonate of soda. Knead into a soft dough.

- Divide the dough into 30 walnut-sized balls. Flatten slightly to form the muthias. Set aside.

- Heat the oil in a saucepan. Add the ajowan seeds, mustard seeds and asafoetida. Let them splutter for 15 seconds.

- Add the muthias and water.

- Cover with a lid and simmer for 10-15 minutes. Serve hot.

Pumpkin Koot

(Pumpkin in Lentil Curry)

Serves 4

Ingredients

50g/1¾oz fresh coconut, grated

1 tsp cumin seeds

2 red chillies

150g/5½oz mung dhal*, soaked for 30 minutes and drained

2 tbsp chana dhal*

Salt to taste

500ml/16fl oz water

2 tbsp refined vegetable oil

250g/9oz pumpkin, diced

¼ tsp turmeric

Method

- Grind the coconut, cumin seeds and red chillies to a paste. Set aside.

- Mix the dhals with the salt and water. Cook this mixture in a saucepan on a medium heat for 40 minutes. Set aside.

- Heat the oil in a saucepan. Add the pumpkin, turmeric, boiled dhals and the coconut paste. Mix well. Simmer for 10 minutes. Serve hot.

Rassa

(Cauliflower and Peas in Sauce)

Serves 4

Ingredients

2 tbsp refined vegetable oil plus extra for deep frying

250g/9oz cauliflower florets

2 tbsp fresh coconut, grated

1cm/½in root ginger, crushed

4-5 green chillies, slit lengthways

2-3 tomatoes, finely chopped

400g/14oz frozen peas

1 tsp sugar

Salt to taste

Method

- Heat the oil for deep frying in a saucepan. Add the cauliflower. Deep fry on a medium heat till golden brown. Drain and set aside.

- Grind the coconut, ginger, green chillies and tomatoes. Heat 2 tbsp oil in a saucepan. Add this paste and fry for 1-2 minutes.

- Add the cauliflower and the remaining ingredients. Mix well. Cook on a low heat for 4-5 minutes. Serve hot.

Doodhi Manpasand

(Bottle Gourd in Sauce)

Serves 4

Ingredients

3 tbsp refined vegetable oil

3 dried red chillies

1 large onion, finely chopped

500g/1lb 2oz bottle gourd*, chopped

¼ tsp turmeric

2 tsp ground coriander

1 tsp ground cumin

½ tsp chilli powder

½ tsp garam masala

2.5cm/1in root ginger, finely chopped

2 tomatoes, finely chopped

1 green pepper, cored, deseeded and finely chopped

Salt to taste

2 tsp coriander leaves, finely chopped

Method

- Heat the oil in a saucepan. Fry the red chillies and onion for 2 minutes.
- Add the remaining ingredients, except the coriander leaves. Mix well. Cook on a low heat for 5-7 minutes. Garnish with the coriander leaves. Serve hot.

Tomato Chokha

(Tomato Compote)

Serves 4

Ingredients

6 large tomatoes

2 tbsp refined vegetable oil

1 big onion, finely chopped

8 garlic cloves, finely chopped

1 green chilli, finely chopped

½ tsp chilli powder

10g/¼oz coriander leaves, finely chopped

Salt to taste

Method

- Grill the tomatoes for 10 minutes. Peel and crush to a pulp. Set aside.
- Heat the oil in a saucepan. Add the onion, garlic and green chilli. Fry for 2-3 minutes. Add the remaining ingredients and the tomato pulp. Mix well. Cover with a lid and cook for 5-6 minutes. Serve hot.

Baingan Chokha

(Aubergine Compote)

Serves 4

Ingredients

1 large aubergine

2 tbsp refined vegetable oil

1 small onion, chopped

8 garlic cloves, finely chopped

1 green chilli, finely chopped

1 tomato, finely chopped

60g/2oz corn kernels, boiled

10g/¼oz coriander leaves, finely chopped

Salt to taste

Method

- Pierce the aubergine all over with a fork. Grill for 10-15 minutes. Peel and crush to a pulp. Set aside.
- Heat the oil in a saucepan. Add the onion, garlic and green chilli. Fry them on a medium heat for 5 minutes.
- Add the remaining ingredients and the aubergine pulp. Mix well. Cook for 3-4 minutes. Serve hot.

Cauliflower & Peas Curry

Serves 4

Ingredients

3 tbsp refined vegetable oil

¼ tsp turmeric

3 green chillies, slit lengthways

1 tsp ground coriander

2.5cm/1in root ginger, grated

250g/9oz cauliflower florets

400g/14oz fresh green peas

60ml/2fl oz water

Salt to taste

1 tbsp coriander leaves, finely chopped

Method

- Heat the oil in a saucepan. Add the turmeric, green chillies, ground coriander and ginger. Fry on a medium heat for a minute.
- Add the remaining ingredients, except the coriander leaves. Mix well Simmer for 10 minutes.
- Garnish with the coriander leaves. Serve hot.

Aloo Methi ki Sabzi

(Potato and Fenugreek Curry)

Serves 4

Ingredients

100g/3½oz fenugreek leaves, chopped

Salt to taste

4 tbsp refined vegetable oil

1 tsp cumin seeds

5-6 green chillies

¼ tsp turmeric

Pinch of asafoetida

6 large potatoes, boiled and chopped

Method

- Mix the fenugreek leaves with the salt. Set aside for 10 minutes.
- Heat the oil in a saucepan. Add the cumin seeds, chillies and turmeric. Let them splutter for 15 seconds.
- Add the remaining ingredients and the fenugreek leaves. Mix well. Cook for 8-10 minutes on a low heat. Serve hot.

Sweet & Sour Karela

Serves 4

Ingredients

500g/1lb 2oz bitter gourds*

Salt to taste

750ml/1¼ pints water

1cm/½in root ginger

10 garlic cloves

4 large onions, chopped

4 tbsp refined vegetable oil

Pinch of asafoetida

½ tsp turmeric

1 tsp ground coriander

1 tsp ground cumin

1 tsp tamarind paste

2 tbsp jaggery*, grated

Method

- Peel the bitter gourds. Slice and soak them in salty water for 1 hour. Rinse and squeeze out the excess water. Wash and set aside.

- Grind the ginger, garlic and onions to a paste. Set aside.

- Heat the oil in a saucepan. Add the asafoetida. Let it splutter for 15 seconds. Add the ginger-onion paste and the remaining ingredients. Mix well. Fry for 3-4 minutes. Add the bitter gourds. Mix well. Cover with a lid and cook on a low heat for 8-10 minutes. Serve hot.

Karela Koshimbir

(Crispy Crushed Bitter Gourd)

Serves 4

Ingredients

500g/1lb 2oz bitter gourds*, peeled

Salt to taste

Refined vegetable oil for frying

2 medium-sized onions, chopped

50g/1¾oz coriander leaves, chopped

3 green chillies, finely chopped

½ fresh coconut, grated

1 tbsp lemon juice

Method

- Slice the bitter gourds. Rub the salt on them and set aside for 2-3 hours.
- Heat the oil in a saucepan. Add the bitter gourds and fry on a medium heat till brown and crispy. Drain, cool a little and crush with your fingers.
- Mix the remaining ingredients in a bowl. Add the gourds and serve while they are still warm.

Karela Curry

(Bitter Gourd Curry)

Serves 4

Ingredients

½ coconut

2 red chillies

1 tsp cumin seeds

3 tbsp refined vegetable oil

1 pinch of asafoetida

2 large onions, finely chopped

2 green chillies, finely chopped

Salt to taste

½ tsp turmeric

500g/1lb 2oz bitter gourds*, peeled and chopped

2 tomatoes, finely chopped

Method

- Grate half of the coconut and chop the rest. Set aside.
- Dry roast (see <u>cooking techniques</u>) the grated coconut, red chillies and cumin seeds. Cool and grind together to a fine paste. Set aside.
- Heat the oil in a frying pan. Add the asafoetida, onions, green chillies, salt, turmeric and chopped coconut. Fry for 3 minutes, stirring frequently.
- Add the bitter gourds and tomatoes. Cook for 3-4 minutes.
- Add the ground coconut paste. Cook for 5-7 minutes and serve hot.

Chilli Cauliflower

Serves 4

Ingredients

3 tbsp refined vegetable oil

5cm/2in root ginger, finely chopped

12 garlic cloves, finely chopped

1 cauliflower, chopped into florets

5 red chillies, quartered and deseeded

6 spring onions, halved

3 tomatoes, blanched and chopped

Salt to taste

Method

- Heat the oil in a saucepan. Add the ginger and garlic. Fry on a medium heat for a minute.
- Add the cauliflower and red chillies. Stir-fry for 5 minutes.
- Add the remaining ingredients. Mix well. Cook on a low heat for 7-8 minutes. Serve hot.

Nutty Curry

Serves 4

Ingredients

4 tbsp ghee

10g/¼oz cashew nuts

10g/¼oz almonds, blanched

10-12 peanuts

5-6 raisins

10 pistachios

10 walnuts, chopped

2.5cm/1in root ginger, grated

6 garlic cloves, crushed

4 small onions, finely chopped

4 tomatoes, finely chopped

4 dates, de-seeded and sliced

½ tsp turmeric

125g/4½oz khoya*

1 tsp garam masala

Salt to taste

75g/2½ Cheddar cheese, grated

1 tbsp coriander leaves, chopped

Method

- Heat the ghee in a frying pan. Add all the nuts and fry them on a medium heat till they turn golden brown. Drain and set aside.
- In the same ghee, fry the ginger, garlic and onion till brown.
- Add the fried nuts and all the remaining ingredients, except the cheese and coriander leaves. Cover with a lid. Cook on a low heat for 5 minutes.
- Garnish with the cheese and coriander leaves. Serve hot.

Daikon Leaves Bhaaji

Serves 4

Ingredients

2 tbsp refined vegetable oil

¼ tsp ground cumin

2 red chillies, broken into bits

Pinch of asafoetida

400g/14oz daikon leaves*, chopped

300g/10oz chana dhal*, soaked for 1 hour

1 tsp jaggery*, grated

¼ tsp turmeric

Salt to taste

Method

- Heat the oil in a saucepan. Add the cumin, red chillies and asafoetida.
- Let them splutter for 15 seconds. Add the remaining ingredients. Mix well. Cook on a low heat for 10-15 minutes. Serve hot.

Chhole Aloo

(Chickpea and Potato Curry)

Serves 4

Ingredients

500g/1lb 2oz chickpeas, soaked overnight

Pinch of bicarbonate of soda

Salt to taste

1 litre/1¾ pints water

3 tbsp ghee

2.5cm/1in root ginger, julienned

2 large onions, grated, plus 1 small onion, sliced

2 tomatoes, diced

1 tsp garam masala

1 tsp ground cumin, dry roasted (see <u>cooking techniques</u>)

½ tsp ground green cardamom

½ tsp turmeric

2 large potatoes, boiled and diced

2 tsp tamarind paste

1 tbsp coriander leaves, chopped

Method

- Cook the chickpeas with the bicarbonate of soda, salt and water in a saucepan on a medium heat for 45 minutes. Drain and set aside.
- Heat the ghee in a saucepan. Add the ginger and grated onions. Fry till translucent. Add the remaining ingredients, except the coriander leaves and sliced onion. Mix well. Add the chickpeas and cook for 7-8 minutes.
- Garnish with the coriander leaves and sliced onion. Serve hot.

Peanut Curry

Serves 4

Ingredients

1 tsp poppy seeds

1 tsp coriander seeds

1 tsp cumin seeds

2 red chillies

25g/scant 1oz fresh coconut, grated

3 tbsp ghee

2 small onions, grated

900g/2lb peanuts, pounded

1 tsp amchoor*

½ tsp turmeric

1 big tomato, blanched and chopped

2 tsp jaggery*, grated

500ml/16fl oz water

Salt to taste

15g/½oz coriander leaves, chopped

Method

- Grind the poppy seeds, coriander seeds, cumin seeds, red chillies and coconut to a fine paste. Set aside.
- Heat the ghee in a saucepan. Add the onions. Fry till translucent.
- Add the ground paste and the remaining ingredients, except the coriander leaves. Mix well. Simmer for 7-8 minutes.
- Garnish with the coriander leaves. Serve hot.

French Beans Upkari

(French Beans with Coconut)

Serves 4

Ingredients

1 tbsp refined vegetable oil

½ tsp mustard seeds

½ tsp urad dhal*

2-3 red chillies, broken

500g/1lb 2oz French beans, chopped

1 tsp jaggery*, grated

Salt to taste

25g/scant 1oz fresh coconut, grated

Method

- Heat the oil in a saucepan. Add the mustard seeds. Let them splutter for 15 seconds.
- Add the dhal. Fry till golden brown. Add the remaining ingredients, except the coconut. Mix well. Cook on a low heat for 8-10 minutes.
- Garnish with the coconut. Serve hot.

Karatey Ambadey

(Bitter Gourd and Unripe Mango Curry)

Serves 4

Ingredients

250g/9oz bitter gourd*, sliced

Salt to taste

60g/2oz jaggery*, grated

1 tsp refined vegetable oil

4 dry red chillies

1 tsp urad dhal*

1 tsp fenugreek seeds

2 tsp coriander seeds

50g/1¾oz fresh coconut, grated

¼ tsp turmeric

4 small unripe mangoes

Method

- Rub the bitter gourd pieces with the salt. Set aside for an hour.
- Squeeze out the water from the gourd pieces. Cook them in a saucepan with the jaggery on a medium heat for 4-5 minutes. Set aside.
- Heat the oil in a saucepan. Add the red chillies, dhal, fenugreek and coriander seeds. Fry for a minute. Add the bitter gourd and the remaining ingredients. Mix well. Cook on a low heat for 4-5 minutes. Serve hot.

Kadhai Paneer

(Spicy Paneer)

Serves 4

Ingredients

2 tbsp refined vegetable oil

1 large onion, sliced

3 large green peppers, finely chopped

500g/1lb 2oz paneer*, chopped into 2.5cm/1in pieces

1 tomato, finely chopped

¼ tsp ground coriander, dry roasted (see <u>cooking techniques</u>)

Salt to taste

10g/¼oz coriander leaves, chopped

Method

- Heat the oil in a saucepan. Add the onion and peppers. Fry on a medium heat for 2-3 minutes.
- Add the remaining ingredients, except the coriander leaves. Mix well. Cook on a low heat for 5 minutes. Garnish with the coriander leaves. Serve hot.

Kathirikkai Vangi

(South Indian Aubergine Curry)

Serves 4

Ingredients

150g/5½oz masoor dhal*

Salt to taste

¼ tsp turmeric

500ml/16fl oz water

250g/9oz thin aubergines, sliced

1 tsp refined vegetable oil

¼ tsp mustard seeds

1 tsp tamarind paste

8-10 curry leaves

1 tsp sambhar powder*

Method

- Mix the masoor dhal with salt, a pinch of turmeric and half the water. Cook in a saucepan on a medium heat for 40 minutes. Set aside.

- Cook the aubergines with salt and the remaining turmeric and water in another saucepan on a medium heat for 20 minutes. Set aside.

- Heat the oil in a saucepan. Add the mustard seeds. Let them splutter for 15 seconds. Add the remaining ingredients, the dhal and the aubergine. Mix well. Simmer for 6-7 minutes. Serve hot.

Pitla

(Spicy Gram Flour Curry)

Serves 4

Ingredients

250g/9oz besan*

500ml/16fl oz water

2 tbsp refined vegetable oil

¼ tsp mustard seeds

2 large onions, finely chopped

6 garlic cloves, crushed

2 tbsp tamarind paste

1 tsp garam masala

Salt to taste

1 tbsp coriander leaves, chopped

Method

- Mix the besan and the water. Set aside.
- Heat the oil in a saucepan. Add the mustard seeds. Let them splutter for 15 seconds. Add the onions and garlic. Fry till the onions are brown.
- Add the besan paste. Cook on a low heat till it starts to boil.
- Add the remaining ingredients. Simmer for 5 minutes. Serve hot.

Cauliflower Masala

Serves 4

Ingredients

1 large cauliflower, parboiled (see <u>cooking techniques</u>) in salted water

3 tbsp refined vegetable oil

2 tbsp coriander leaves, finely chopped

1 tsp ground coriander

½ tsp ground cumin

¼ tsp ground ginger

Salt to taste

120ml/4fl oz water

For the sauce:

200g/7oz yoghurt

1 tbsp besan<u>*</u>, dry roasted (see <u>cooking techniques</u>)

¾ tsp chilli powder

Method

- Drain the cauliflower and chop into florets.
- Heat 2 tbsp oil in a frying pan. Add the cauliflower and fry it on a medium heat till golden brown. Set aside.
- Mix all the sauce ingredients together.
- Heat 1 tbsp oil in a saucepan and add this mixture. Fry for a minute.
- Cover with a lid and simmer for 8-10 minutes.
- Add the cauliflower. Mix well. Simmer for 5 minutes.
- Garnish with the coriander leaves. Serve hot.

Shukna Kacha Pepe

(Green Papaya Curry)

Serves 4

Ingredients

150g/5½oz chana dhal*, soaked overnight, drained and ground to a paste

3 tbsp refined vegetable oil plus for deep frying

2 whole dry red chillies

½ tsp fenugreek seeds

½ tsp mustard seeds

1 unripe papaya, peeled and grated

1 tsp turmeric

1 tbsp sugar

Salt to taste

Method

- Divide the dhal paste into walnut-sized balls. Flatten into thin discs.
- Heat the oil for deep frying in a frying pan. Add the discs. Deep fry on a medium heat till golden brown. Drain and break into small pieces. Set aside.
- Heat the remaining oil in a saucepan. Add the chillies, fenugreek and mustard seeds. Let them splutter for 15 seconds.
- Add the remaining ingredients. Mix well. Cover with a lid and cook on a low heat for 8-10 minutes. Add the dhal pieces. Mix well and serve.

Dry Okra

Ingredients

3 tbsp mustard oil

½ tsp kalonji seeds*

750g/1lb 10oz okra, slit lengthways

Salt to taste

½ tsp chilli powder

½ tsp turmeric

2 tsp sugar

3 tsp ground mustard

1 tbsp tamarind paste

Method

- Heat the oil in a saucepan. Fry the onion seeds and okra for 5 minutes.
- Add the salt, chilli powder, turmeric and sugar. Cover with a lid. Cook on a low heat for 10 minutes.
- Add the remaining ingredients. Mix well. Cook for 2-3 minutes. Serve hot.

Moghlai Cauliflower

Ingredients

5cm/2in root ginger

2 tsp cumin seeds

6-7 black peppercorns

500g/1lb 2oz cauliflower florets

Salt to taste

2 tbsp ghee

2 bay leaves

200g/7oz yoghurt

500ml/16fl oz coconut milk

1 tsp sugar

Method

- Grind the ginger, cumin seeds and peppercorns to a fine paste.
- Marinate the cauliflower florets with this paste and salt for 20 minutes.
- Heat the ghee in a frying pan. Add the florets. Fry till golden brown. Add the remaining ingredients. Mix well. Cover with a lid and simmer for 7-8 minutes. Serve hot.

Bhapa Shorshe Baingan

(Aubergine in Mustard Sauce)

Serves 4

Ingredients

2 long aubergines

Salt to taste

¼ tsp turmeric

3 tbsp refined vegetable oil

3 tbsp mustard oil

2–3 tbsp ready-made mustard

1 tbsp coriander leaves, finely chopped

1-2 green chillies, finely chopped

Method

- Slice each aubergine lengthways into 8-12 pieces. Marinate with the salt and turmeric for 5 minutes.
- Heat the oil in a saucepan. Add the aubergine slices and cover with a lid. Cook on a medium heat for 3-4 minutes, turning occasionally.
- Whisk the mustard oil with the ready-made mustard and add to the aubergines. Mix well. Cook on a medium heat for a minute.
- Garnish with the coriander leaves and green chillies. Serve hot.

Baked Vegetables in Spicy Sauce

Serves 4

Ingredients

2 tbsp butter

4 garlic cloves, finely chopped

1 large onion, finely chopped

1 tbsp plain white flour

200g/7oz frozen mixed vegetables

Salt to taste

1 tsp chilli powder

1 tsp mustard paste

250ml/8fl oz ketchup

4 large potatoes, boiled and sliced

250ml/8fl oz white sauce

4 tbsp grated Cheddar cheese

Method

- Heat the butter in a saucepan. Add the garlic and onion. Fry till translucent. Add the flour and fry for a minute.
- Add the vegetables, salt, chilli powder, mustard paste and ketchup. Cook on a medium heat for 4-5 minutes. Set aside.
- Grease a baking dish. Arrange the vegetable mixture and the potatoes in alternate layers. Pour the white sauce and cheese on top.
- Bake in an oven at 200°C (400°F, Gas Mark 6) for 20 minutes. Serve hot.

Tasty Tofu

Serves 4

Ingredients

2 tbsp refined vegetable oil

3 small onions, grated

1 tsp ginger paste

1 tsp garlic paste

3 tomatoes, puréed

50g/1¾oz Greek yoghurt, whisked

400g/14oz tofu, chopped into 2.5cm/1in pieces

25g/scant 1oz coriander leaves, finely chopped

Salt to taste

Method

- Heat the oil in a saucepan. Add the onions, ginger paste and garlic paste. Stir-fry for 5 minutes on a medium heat.
- Add the remaining ingredients. Mix well. Simmer for 3-4 minutes. Serve hot.

Aloo Baingan

(Potato and Aubergine Curry)

Serves 4

Ingredients

3 tbsp refined vegetable oil

1 tsp mustard seeds

½ tsp asafoetida

1cm/½in root ginger, finely chopped

4 green chillies, slit lengthways

10 garlic cloves, finely chopped

6 curry leaves

½ tsp turmeric

3 large potatoes, boiled and diced

250g/9oz aubergines, chopped

½ tsp amchoor*

Salt to taste

Method

- Heat the oil in a saucepan. Add the mustard seeds and asafoetida. Let them splutter for 15 seconds.
- Add the ginger, green chillies, garlic and curry leaves. Fry for 1 minute, stirring continuously.
- Add the remaining ingredients. Mix well. Cover with a lid and simmer for 10-12 minutes. Serve hot.

Sugar Snap Pea Curry

Serves 4

Ingredients

500g/1lb 2oz sugar snap peas

2 tbsp refined vegetable oil

1 tsp ginger paste

1 large onion, finely chopped

2 large potatoes, peeled and diced

½ tsp turmeric

½ tsp garam masala

½ tsp chilli powder

1 tsp sugar

2 large tomatoes, diced

Salt to taste

Method

- Peel the strings from the edges of the pea pods. Chop the pods. Set aside.
- Heat the oil in a saucepan. Add the ginger paste and onion. Fry till translucent. Add the remaining ingredients and the pods. Mix well. Cover with a lid and cook on a low heat for 7-8 minutes. Serve hot.

Potato Pumpkin Curry

Serves 4

Ingredients

2 tbsp refined vegetable oil

1 tsp panch phoron*

Pinch of asafoetida

1 dried red chilli, broken into bits

1 bay leaf

4 large potatoes, diced

200g/7oz pumpkin, diced

½ tsp ginger paste

½ tsp garlic paste

1 tsp ground cumin

1 tsp ground coriander

¼ tsp turmeric

½ tsp garam masala

1 tsp amchoor*

500ml/16fl oz water

Salt to taste

Method

- Heat the oil in a saucepan. Add the panch phoron. Let them splutter for 15 seconds.
- Add the asafoetida, red chilli pieces and the bay leaf. Fry for a minute.
- Add the remaining ingredients. Mix well. Simmer for 10-12 minutes. Serve hot.

Egg Thoran

(Spicy Scrambled Egg)

Serves 4

Ingredients

60ml/2fl oz refined vegetable oil

¼ tsp mustard seeds

2 onions, finely chopped

1 large tomato, finely chopped

1 tsp freshly ground black pepper

Salt to taste

4 eggs, whisked

25g/scant 1oz fresh coconut, grated

50g/1¾oz coriander leaves, chopped

Method

- Heat the oil in a saucepan and fry the mustard seeds. Let them splutter for 15 seconds. Add the onions and fry till brown. Add the tomato, pepper and salt. Fry for 2-3 minutes.
- Add the eggs. Cook on a low heat, scrambling continuously.
- Garnish with the coconut and coriander leaves. Serve hot.

Baingan Lajawab

(Aubergine with Cauliflower)

Serves 4

Ingredients

4 large aubergines

2 tbsp refined vegetable oil plus extra for deep frying

1 tsp cumin seeds

½ tsp turmeric

2.5cm/1in root ginger, ground

2 green chillies, finely chopped

1 tsp amchoor*

Salt to taste

100g/3½oz frozen peas

Method

- Slit each aubergine lengthways and scoop out the flesh.
- Heat the oil. Add the aubergine shells. Deep fry for 2 minutes. Set aside.
- Heat 2 tbsp oil in a saucepan. Add the cumin seeds and turmeric. Let them splutter for 15 seconds. Add the remaining ingredients and the aubergine flesh. Mash lightly and cook on a low heat for 5 minutes.
- Carefully stuff the aubergine shells with this mixture. Grill for 3-4 minutes. Serve hot.

Veggie Bahar

(Vegetables in a Nutty Sauce)

Serves 4

Ingredients

3 tbsp refined vegetable oil

1 large onion, finely chopped

2 large tomatoes, finely chopped

1 tsp ginger paste

1 tsp garlic paste

20 cashew nuts, ground

2 tbsp walnuts, ground

2 tbsp poppy seeds

200g/7oz yoghurt

100g/3½oz frozen mixed vegetables

1 tsp garam masala

Salt to taste

Method

- Heat the oil in a saucepan. Add the onion. Fry on a medium heat till brown. Add the tomatoes, ginger paste, garlic paste, cashew nuts, walnuts and poppy seeds. Fry for 3-4 minutes.
- Add the remaining ingredients. Cook for 7-8 minutes. Serve hot.

Stuffed Vegetables

Serves 4

Ingredients

4 small potatoes

100g/3½oz okra

4 small aubergines

4 tbsp refined vegetable oil

½ tsp mustard seeds

Pinch of asafoetida

For the filling:

250g/9oz besan*

1 tsp ground coriander

1 tsp ground cumin

½ tsp turmeric

1 tsp chilli powder

1 tsp garam masala

Salt to taste

Method

- Mix all the filling ingredients together. Set aside.
- Slit the potatoes, okra and aubergines. Stuff with the filling. Set aside.
- Heat the oil in a saucepan. Add the mustard seeds and asafoetida. Let them splutter for 15 seconds. Add the stuffed vegetables. Cover with a lid and cook on a low heat for 8-10 minutes. Serve hot.

Singhi Aloo

(Drumsticks with Potatoes)

Serves 4

Ingredients

5 tbsp refined vegetable oil

3 small onions, finely chopped

3 green chillies, finely chopped

2 large tomatoes, finely chopped

2 tsp ground coriander

Salt to taste

5 Indian drumsticks*, chopped into 7.5cm/3in pieces

2 large potatoes, chopped

360ml/12fl oz water

Method

- Heat the oil in a saucepan. Add the onions and chillies. Fry them on a low heat for a minute.
- Add the tomatoes, ground coriander and salt. Fry for 2-3 minutes.
- Add the drumsticks, potatoes and water. Mix well. Simmer for 10-12 minutes. Serve hot.

Sindhi Curry

Serves 4

Ingredients

150g/5½oz masoor dhal*

Salt to taste

1 litre/1¾ pints water

4 tomatoes, finely chopped

5 tbsp refined vegetable oil

½ tsp cumin seeds

¼ tsp fenugreek seeds

8 curry leaves

3 green chillies, slit lengthways

¼ tsp asafoetida

4 tbsp besan*

½ tsp chilli powder

½ tsp turmeric

8 okras, slit lengthways

10 French beans, diced

6-7 kokum*

1 large carrot, julienned

1 large potato, diced

Method

- Mix the dhal with the salt and water. Cook this mixture in a saucepan on a medium heat for 45 minutes, stirring occasionally.
- Add the tomatoes and simmer for 7-8 minutes. Set aside.
- Heat the oil in a saucepan. Add the cumin and fenugreek seeds, curry leaves, green chillies and asafoetida. Let them splutter for 30 seconds.
- Add the besan. Fry for a minute, stirring constantly.
- Add the remaining ingredients and the dhal mixture. Mix thoroughly. Simmer for 10 minutes. Serve hot.

Gulnar Kofta

(Paneer Balls In Spinach)

Ingredients

150g/5½oz mixed dry fruits

200g/7oz khoya*

4 large potatoes, boiled and mashed

150g/5½oz paneer*, crumbled

100g/3½oz Cheddar cheese

2 tsp cornflour

Refined vegetable oil for deep frying

2 tsp butter

100g/3½oz spinach, finely chopped

1 tsp single cream

Salt to taste

For the spice mixture:

2 cloves

1cm/½in cinnamon

3 black peppercorns

Method

- Mix the dry fruits with the khoya. Set aside.
- Grind together all the ingredients of the spice mixture. Set aside.
- Mix the potatoes, paneer, cheese and cornflour into a dough. Divide the dough into walnut-sized balls and flatten into discs. Place a portion of the dry fruit-khoya mixture on each disc and seal like a pouch.
- Smooth into walnut-sized balls to make the koftas. Set aside.
- Heat the oil in a frying pan. Add the koftas and deep fry them on a medium heat till they turn golden brown. Drain and set aside in a serving dish.
- Heat the butter in a saucepan. Add the ground spice mixture. Fry for a minute.
- Add the spinach and cook for 2-3 minutes.
- Add the cream and salt. Mix well. Pour this mixture over the koftas. Serve hot.

Paneer Korma

(Rich Paneer Curry)

Serves 4

Ingredients

500g/1lb 2oz paneer*

3 tbsp refined vegetable oil

1 large onion, chopped

2.5cm/1in root ginger, julienned

8 garlic cloves, crushed

2 green chillies, finely chopped

1 large tomato, finely chopped

¼ tsp turmeric

½ tsp ground coriander

½ tsp ground cumin

1 tsp chilli powder

½ tsp garam masala

125g/4½oz yoghurt

Salt to taste

250ml/8fl oz water

2 tbsp coriander leaves, finely chopped

Method

- Grate half of the paneer and chop the remainder into 2.5cm/1in pieces.
- Heat the oil in a frying pan. Add the paneer pieces. Fry them on a medium heat till they turn golden brown. Drain and set aside.
- In the same oil, fry the onion, ginger, garlic and green chillies on a medium heat for 2-3 minutes.
- Add the tomato. Fry for 2 minutes.
- Add the turmeric, ground coriander, ground cumin, chilli powder and garam masala. Mix well. Fry for 2-3 minutes.
- Add the yoghurt, salt and water. Mix well. Simmer for 8-10 minutes.
- Add the fried paneer pieces. Mix well. Simmer for 5 minutes.
- Garnish with the grated paneer and coriander leaves. Serve hot.

Chutney Potatoes

Serves 4

Ingredients

100g/3½oz coriander leaves, finely chopped

4 green chillies

2.5cm/1in root ginger

7 garlic cloves

25g/scant 1oz fresh coconut, grated

1 tbsp lemon juice

1 tsp cumin seeds

1 tsp coriander seeds

½ tsp turmeric

½ tsp chilli powder

Salt to taste

750g/1lb 10oz large potatoes, peeled and chopped into discs

4 tbsp refined vegetable oil

¼ tsp mustard seeds

Method

- Mix the coriander leaves, green chillies, ginger, garlic, coconut, lemon juice, cumin and coriander seeds. Grind this mixture to a fine paste.
- Mix this paste with the turmeric, chilli powder and salt.
- Marinate the potatoes with this mixture for 30 minutes.
- Heat the oil in a saucepan. Add the mustard seeds. Let them splutter for 15 seconds.
- Add the potatoes. Cook them on a low heat for 8-10 minutes, stirring occasionally. Serve hot.

Lobia

(Black Eyed Peas Curry)

Ingredients

400g/14oz black eyed peas, soaked overnight

Pinch of bicarbonate of soda

Salt to taste

1.4 litres/2½ pints water

1 large onion

4 garlic cloves

3 tbsp ghee

2 tsp ground coriander

1 tsp ground cumin

1 tsp amchoor*

½ tsp garam masala

½ tsp chilli powder

¼ tsp turmeric

2 tomatoes, diced

3 green chillies, finely chopped

2 tbsp coriander leaves,

finely chopped

Method

- Mix the black eyed peas with the bicarbonate of soda, salt and 1.2 litres/2 pints of water. Cook this mixture in a saucepan on a medium heat for 45 minutes. Drain and set aside.
- Grind the onion and garlic to a paste.
- Heat the ghee in a saucepan. Add the paste and fry it on a medium heat till it turns brown.
- Add the cooked black eyed peas, the remaining water and all the remaining ingredients, except the coriander leaves. Simmer for 8-10 minutes.
- Garnish with the coriander leaves. Serve hot.

Khatta Meetha Vegetable

(Sweet and Sour Vegetables)

Serves 4

Ingredients

1 tbsp flour

1 tbsp malt vinegar

2 tbsp sugar

50g/1¾oz cabbage, finely chopped into long strips

1 large green pepper, chopped into strips

1 large carrot, chopped into strips

50g/1¾oz French beans, slit and chopped

100g/3½oz baby corn

1 tbsp refined vegetable oil

½ tsp ginger paste

½ tsp garlic paste

2-3 green chillies, finely chopped

4-5 spring onions, finely chopped

125g/4½oz tomato purée

120ml/8fl oz ketchup

Salt to taste

10g/¼oz coriander leaves, finely chopped

Method

- Mix the flour with the vinegar and sugar. Set aside.
- Mix together the cabbage, green pepper, carrot, French beans and baby corn. Steam (see <u>cooking techniques</u>) this mixture in a steamer for 10 minutes. Set aside.
- Heat the oil in a saucepan. Add the ginger paste, garlic paste and chillies. Fry for 30 seconds.
- Add the spring onions. Fry for 1-2 minutes.
- Add the steamed vegetables and the tomato purée, ketchup and salt. Cook on a low heat for 5-6 minutes.
- Add the flour paste. Cook for 3-4 minutes.
- Garnish with the coriander leaves. Serve hot.

Dahiwale Chhole

(Chickpea in Yoghurt Sauce)

Serves 4

Ingredients

500g/1lb 2oz chickpeas, soaked overnight

Pinch of bicarbonate of soda

Salt to taste

1 litre/1¾ pints water

3 tbsp ghee

2 large onions, grated

1 tsp ginger, grated

150g/5½oz yoghurt

1 tsp garam masala

1 tsp ground cumin, dry roasted (see cooking techniques)

½ tsp chilli powder

¼ tsp turmeric

1 tsp amchoor*

½ tbsp cashew nuts

½ tbsp raisins

Method

- Mix the chickpeas with the bicarbonate of soda, salt and water. Cook this mixture in a saucepan on a medium heat for 45 minutes. Drain and set aside.
- Heat the ghee in a saucepan. Add the onions and ginger. Fry them on a medium heat till the onions are translucent.
- Add the chickpeas and the remaining ingredients, except the cashew nuts and raisins. Mix well. Cook on a low heat for 7-8 minutes.
- Garnish with the cashew nuts and raisins. Serve hot.

Teekha Papad Bhaji*

(Spicy Poppadam Dish)

Serves 4

Ingredients

1 tbsp refined vegetable oil

¼ tsp mustard seeds

¼ tsp cumin seeds

¼ tsp fenugreek seeds

2 tsp ground coriander

3 tsp sugar

Salt to taste

250ml/8fl oz water

6 poppadams, broken into bits

1 tbsp coriander leaves, chopped

Method

- Heat the oil in a saucepan. Add the mustard, cumin and fenugreek seeds, ground coriander, sugar and salt. Let them splutter for 30 seconds. Add the water and simmer for 3-4 minutes.
- Add the poppadam pieces. Simmer for 5-7 minutes. Garnish with the coriander leaves. Serve hot.

Paneer Pulao

Serves 4

Ingredients

4 tbsp refined vegetable oil

2 large onions, sliced

1 tsp ginger paste

1 tsp garlic paste

2 green chillies, finely chopped

400g/14oz paneer*, diced

400g/14oz tomato purée

375g/13oz basmati rice

Salt to taste

600ml/1 pint hot water

1 tbsp coriander leaves, chopped

Method

- Heat the oil in a saucepan. Fry the onions, ginger paste, garlic paste and green chillies on a medium heat for 2 minutes, stirring continuously.
- Add the paneer and tomato purée. Cook the mixture for 2-3 minutes.
- Add the rice, salt and water. Cook over a low heat till the rice is cooked.
- Garnish the pulao with the coriander leaves. Serve hot.

Coconut Rice

Ingredients

3 tbsp ghee

1 large onion, finely chopped

6 garlic cloves, finely chopped

2 green cardamom pods

2.5cm/1in cinnamon

2 cloves

4 black peppercorns

300g/10oz basmati rice, soaked for 30 minutes and drained

1.2 litres/2 pints coconut milk

Salt to taste

Method

- Heat the ghee in a saucepan. Add the onion, garlic, cardamom, cinnamon, cloves and peppercorns. Fry them on a medium heat for 3-4 minutes.
- Add the drained rice. Stir-fry on a medium heat for 2-3 minutes.

- Add the coconut milk and salt. Mix well and simmer for 7-8 minutes.
- Cover with a lid and cook for 15 more minutes.
- Serve hot.

Saffron Pulao

Ingredients

4 tbsp ghee

1 tsp cumin seeds

2 bay leaves

375g/13oz basmati rice, soaked for 30 minutes and drained

Salt to taste

750ml/1¼ pints hot water

1 tsp saffron

1 tbsp coriander leaves, finely chopped

Method

- Heat the ghee in a saucepan. Add the cumin seeds and bay leaves. Let them splutter for 15 seconds.
- Add the rice and salt. Fry the mixture on a medium heat for 3-4 minutes.
- Add the hot water and the saffron. Simmer for 8-10 minutes or till the rice is cooked, stirring at regular intervals.
- Garnish with the coriander leaves. Serve hot.

Dhal Rice Mix

Serves 4

Ingredients

2 tbsp masoor dhal*

2 tbsp urad dhal*

2 tbsp mung dhal*

2 tbsp chana dhal*

500ml/16fl oz water

4 tbsp ghee

1 large onion, finely sliced

1 tsp garam masala

250g/9oz basmati rice, parboiled

1 tsp turmeric

1 bay leaf

Salt to taste

250ml/8fl oz milk

Method

- Mix all the dhals together. Cook them with the water in a saucepan on a medium heat for 30 minutes. Set aside.
- Heat the ghee in a saucepan. Add the onion and garam masala. Fry on a medium heat till the onion is translucent.
- Add the rice, turmeric, bay leaf and salt. Mix well. Add the milk and the dhal mixture. Cover with a lid and simmer for 7-8 minutes. Serve hot.

Kairi Bhaat

(Rice with Green Mango)

Serves 4

Ingredients

4 tbsp refined vegetable oil

½ tsp mustard seeds

Pinch of asafoetida

½ tsp turmeric

8 curry leaves

180g/6¼oz roasted peanuts

1 tsp ground coriander

2 unripe mangoes, peeled and grated

Salt to taste

300g/10oz steamed rice

Method

- Heat the oil in a saucepan. Add the mustard seeds, asafoetida, turmeric and curry leaves. Let them splutter for 15 seconds.
- Add the peanuts, ground coriander, mangoes and salt. Fry them on a medium heat for 5 minutes.
- Add the cooked rice and stir the bhaat gently. Serve hot.

Prawn Khichdi

Serves 4

Ingredients

5 tbsp refined vegetable oil

3 small onions, finely chopped

250g/9oz prawns, cleaned and de-veined

1 tsp ginger paste

1 tsp garlic paste

2 tsp ground coriander

1 tsp ground cumin

½ tsp turmeric

375g/13oz long-grained rice

Salt to taste

360ml/12fl oz hot water

360ml/12fl oz coconut milk

Method

- Heat the oil in a saucepan. Fry the onions till translucent.

- Add the prawns, ginger paste, garlic paste, ground coriander, ground cumin and turmeric. Sauté on a medium heat for 3-4 minutes.
- Add the remaining ingredients. Simmer for 10 minutes. Serve hot.

Curd Rice

Serves 4

Ingredients

300g/10oz steamed rice

400g/14oz yoghurt

8-10 curry leaves

3 green chillies, slit lengthways

Pinch of asafoetida

1 tbsp coriander leaves, finely chopped

Salt to taste

2 tsp refined vegetable oil

½ tsp mustard seeds

¼ tsp cumin seeds

½ tsp urad dhal*

Method

- Mash the rice with a wooden spoon. Mix with the yoghurt, curry leaves, green chillies, asafoetida, coriander leaves and salt. Set aside.

- Heat the oil in a saucepan. Add the mustard seeds, cumin seeds and urad dhal. Let them splutter for 15 seconds.

- Pour this mixture directly on top of the rice mixture. Stir thoroughly.

- Serve chilled with hot mango pickle

Chicken & Rice Hotpot

Serves 4

Ingredients

3 tbsp refined vegetable oil

4 cloves

5cm/2in cinnamon

2 green cardamom pods

2 bay leaves

3 large onions, finely chopped

12 chicken drumsticks

½ tsp ginger paste

½ tsp garlic paste

3 chicken stock cubes, dissolved in 1.7 litres/3 pints hot water

½ tsp freshly ground black pepper

Salt to taste

500g/1lb 2oz basmati rice

250g/9oz carrots, thinly sliced

Method

- Heat the oil in a saucepan. Add the cloves, cinnamon, cardamom and bay leaves. Let them splutter for 15 seconds.
- Add the onions. Cook for 2 minutes. Add all the remaining ingredients, except the rice and carrots. Mix well. Cook for 4-5 minutes.
- Add the rice and carrots, and stir well. Cover with a lid and simmer for 35-40 minutes. Serve hot.

Corn Pulao

Serves 4

Ingredients

5 tbsp refined vegetable oil

2 small onions, finely chopped

300g/10oz corn kernels, boiled

2 tsp ground coriander

1 tsp ground cumin

¼ tsp turmeric

125g/4½oz tomato purée

Salt to taste

375g/13oz basmati rice

500ml/16fl oz hot water

1 tsp lemon juice

1 tbsp coriander leaves, chopped

Method

- Heat the oil in a pan. Fry the onions on a medium heat till translucent. Add the remaining ingredients, except the rice, water, lemon juice and coriander. Fry for 3-4 minutes. Add the rice, water and lemon juice.
- Simmer for 10 minutes. Sprinkle coriander leaves on top and serve hot.

Dhansak Rice

(Spicy Parsi Rice)

Serves 4

Ingredients

60ml/2fl oz refined vegetable oil

2 bay leaves

2 green cardamom pods

4 black peppercorns

2.5cm/1in cinnamon

1 tsp sugar

1 large onion, finely chopped

375g/13oz long-grained rice, soaked for 10 minutes and drained

Salt to taste

750ml/1¼ pints hot water

Method

- Heat the oil in a saucepan. Add the bay leaves, cardamom, peppercorns, cinnamon and sugar. Stir on a medium heat till the sugar has caramelized.
- Add the onion and fry on a medium heat till it turns brown. Add the rice and stir until the rice turns brown.

- Add the salt and the hot water. Cover with a lid and cook for 10 minutes over a low heat.
- Serve hot with Dhansak

Brown Rice

Ingredients

3 tbsp refined vegetable oil

½ tsp ginger paste

½ tsp garlic paste

2 large onions, quartered

375g/13oz long-grained rice, soaked for 30 minutes and drained

1 tsp garam masala

600ml/1 pint hot water

Salt to taste

Method

- Heat the oil in a saucepan. Add the ginger paste and garlic paste. Fry for a few seconds.
- Add the onion pieces and sauté them on a medium heat for a minute.
- Add the drained rice and garam masala. Cook for 2-3 minutes, stirring well.
- Add the hot water and salt. Simmer the mixture till the rice is cooked.
- Serve hot.

Lightning Source UK Ltd.
Milton Keynes UK
UKHW021852270521
384511UK00002B/314